QUICK AND HEALTHY VEGETARIAN MEALS FOR TYPE 2 DIABETES

Delicious, Time-Saving Dishes for Blood Sugar Management & Plant-Based Wellness

By Mia Bennett

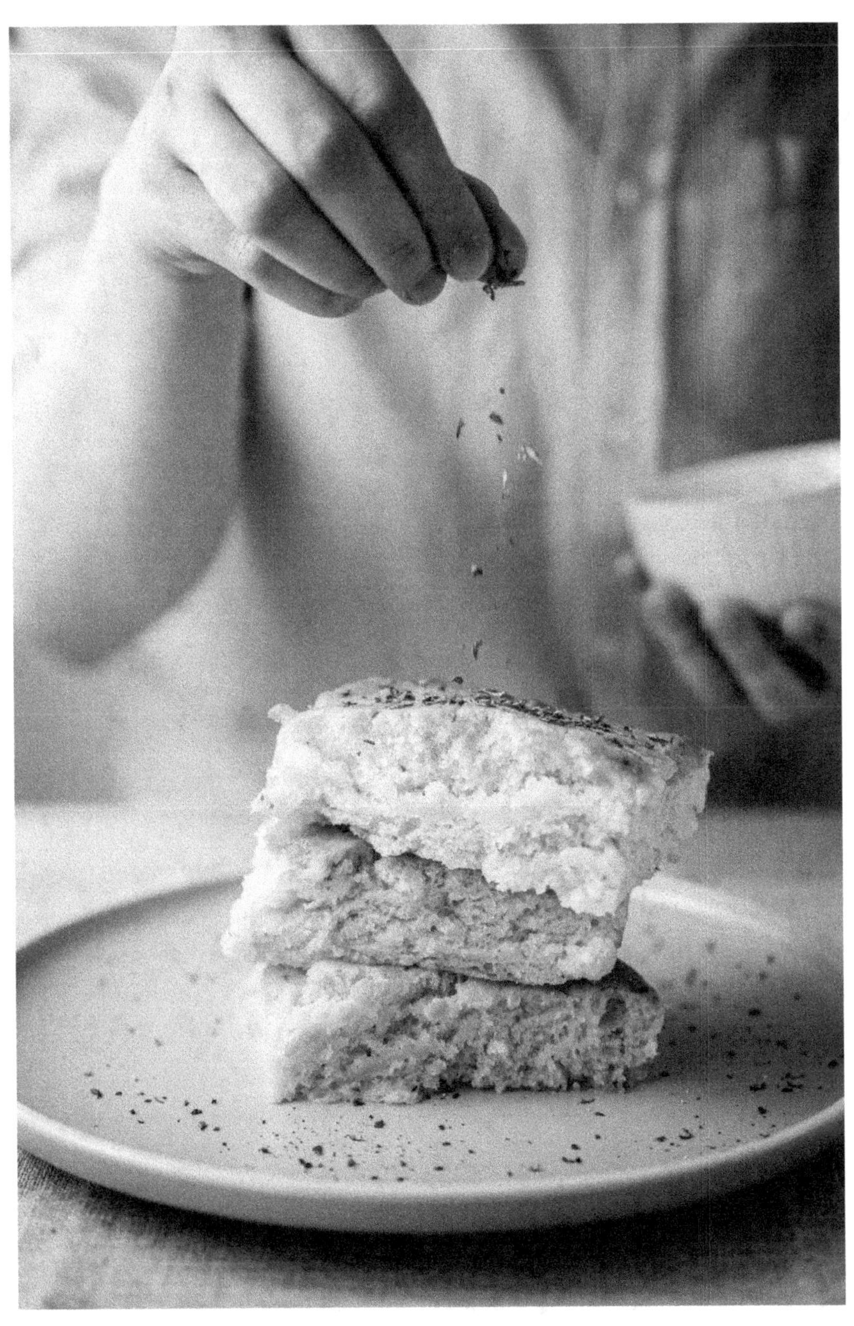

TABLE OF CONTENTS

INTRODUCTION

Type 2 diabetes, a condition where your body struggles to regulate blood sugar, can feel overwhelming. But you're not alone. Millions around the world manage this condition, and a key player in that journey is your diet. Let's delve into understanding Type 2 diabetes, the importance of a balanced diet, how vegetarian meals can be beneficial, and the essential nutrients you need to prioritize.

Understanding Type 2 Diabetes: The Insulin Connection

Imagine your body is a grand house, and sugar is the energy source. Insulin, a hormone, acts like a key that unlocks the doors to your cells, allowing sugar to enter and fuel them. In Type 2 diabetes, either your body doesn't produce enough insulin, or your cells become resistant to its message. This sugar backup in the bloodstream can lead to various health issues.

The Power of a Balanced Plate: Friend, Not Foe

Think of your diet as a beautiful painting. To manage diabetes effectively, you need a balanced canvas. Here's what your masterpiece might include:

- **Vibrant Veggies:** Load up on these colorful wonders. They're packed with vitamins, minerals, and fiber, which helps regulate blood sugar absorption. Leafy greens, broccoli, and peppers are all-stars.
- **Whole Grains:** Ditch the refined white stuff. Opt for brown rice, quinoa, and whole-wheat bread. These complex carbohydrates provide sustained energy without spiking your blood sugar.
- **Lean Protein:** Whether it's fish, beans, or skinless chicken, protein helps with feeling fuller for longer and can aid in weight management, another crucial factor in diabetes control.
- **Healthy Fats**: Don't fear all fats! Avocados, nuts (in moderation), and olive oil are excellent sources of healthy fats that can improve satiety and heart health, often a concern for diabetics.

Why Vegetarian Meals Can Shine

Vegetarian diets tend to be naturally lower in saturated fat and cholesterol, common culprits in heart complications that can arise with diabetes. They're also generally rich in fiber, keeping you feeling full and your blood sugar stable. Here's how to make vegetarian meals work for you:

- **Embrace Legumes**: Beans, lentils, and chickpeas are protein powerhouses that can replace meat in many dishes. They're also high in fiber and some essential vitamins.
- **Eggs for Everyone**: While not strictly vegetarian, eggs are a complete protein source and a versatile ingredient for breakfast, lunch, or dinner.
- **Don't Forget Dairy (if tolerated):** Cheese and yogurt can provide calcium and vitamin D, both important for bone health. Opt for low-fat options and be mindful of portion sizes.

Essential Nutrients: Your Body's Best Friends

Certain nutrients become even more critical when managing diabetes. Here are some to keep on your radar:

- **Chromium**: This mineral helps your body use insulin more effectively. Include broccoli, whole grains, and some meats in your diet.

- **Vitamin D:** Crucial for bone health and may improve insulin sensitivity. Get sunshine, and consider fortified foods like milk.

- **Magnesium**: Plays a role in blood sugar control and nerve function. Leafy greens, nuts, and seeds are good sources.

Remember: This is just a starting point. With the right knowledge and dietary approach, you can turn your plate into a powerful tool for managing your diabetes and living a fulfilling life.

Chapter 1: 30 Day Meal Plan

Week 1

Day 1

- Breakfast: Spinach and Mushroom Breakfast Burrito
- Lunch: Lentil and Vegetable Soup
- Dinner: Spaghetti Squash with Marinara Sauce
- Snack: Hummus with Carrot and Cucumber Sticks
- Dessert: Dark Chocolate Avocado Mousse

Day 2

- Breakfast: Greek Yogurt with Berries and Nuts
- Lunch: Chickpea and Avocado Salad
- Dinner: Baked Tofu with Steamed Vegetables
- Snack: Baked Kale Chips
- Dessert: Baked Apples with Cinnamon

Day 3

- Breakfast: Avocado Toast with Tomato and Basil
- Lunch: Quinoa and Black Bean Stuffed Peppers
- Dinner: Mushroom and Spinach Lasagna
- Snack: Roasted Chickpeas
- Dessert: Chia Seed Pudding with Mango

Day 4

- Breakfast: Chia Seed Pudding with Almond Milk
- Lunch: Grilled Vegetable Wrap
- Dinner: Stuffed Bell Peppers with Quinoa and Vegetables
- Snack: Edamame with Sea Salt
- Dessert: Berry and Greek Yogurt Parfait

Day 5

- Breakfast: Scrambled Tofu with Vegetables
- Lunch: Spinach and Feta Stuffed Portobellos
- Dinner: Vegetable and Bean Enchiladas
- Snack: Stuffed Mini Bell Peppers
- Dessert: Almond Flour Brownies

Day 6

- Breakfast: Overnight Oats with Flaxseeds
- Lunch: Zucchini Noodles with Pesto
- Dinner: Cauliflower Crust Pizza with Veggies
- Snack: Guacamole with Whole Grain Crackers
- Dessert: Banana and Oat Cookies

Day 7

- Breakfast: Veggie-Packed Frittata
- Lunch: Roasted Beet and Arugula Salad

- Dinner: Lentil Shepherd's Pie

- Snack: Almond and Date Energy Balls

- Dessert: Coconut Flour Chocolate Cake

Week 2

Day 8

- Breakfast: Quinoa Breakfast Bowl

- Lunch: Sweet Potato and Lentil Buddha Bowl

- Dinner: Eggplant Stir-Fry with Tofu

- Snack: Veggie Spring Rolls with Peanut Sauce

- Dessert: Mixed Berry Crumble

Day 9

- Breakfast: Smoothie Bowl with Fresh Fruits

- Lunch: Vegetable Stir-Fry with Brown Rice

- Dinner: Zucchini and Corn Tacos

- Snack: Greek Yogurt Dip with Veggies

- Dessert: Frozen Yogurt Bark with Berries

Day 10

- Breakfast: Whole Grain Pancakes with Berry Compote

- Lunch: Tomato Basil Soup with Whole Grain Bread

- Dinner: Vegetable Paella

- Snack: Caprese Salad Skewers

- Dessert: Apple Cinnamon Muffins

Day 11

- Breakfast: Sweet Potato and Black Bean Hash

- Lunch: Cauliflower Rice Burrito Bowl

- Dinner: Grilled Vegetable Skewers with Couscous

- Snack: Spicy Roasted Cauliflower Bites

- Dessert: Carrot Cake Energy Balls

Day 12

- Breakfast: Cottage Cheese with Pineapple and Walnuts

- Lunch: Mediterranean Chickpea Salad

- Dinner: Moroccan Chickpea Stew

- Snack: Avocado and Bean Dip

- Dessert: Peach Sorbet

Day 13

- Breakfast: Almond Butter Banana Sandwich

- Lunch: Tofu and Broccoli Salad with Peanut Dressing

- Dinner: Spinach and Ricotta Stuffed Shells

- Snack: Mini Quinoa Patties

- Dessert: Sugar-Free Lemon Bars

Day 14

- Breakfast: Berry and Spinach Smoothie
- Lunch: Mixed Bean Chili
- Dinner: Broccoli and Tofu Stir-Fry
- Snack: Apple Slices with Almond Butter
- Dessert: Pumpkin Spice Bites

Week 3

Day 15

- Breakfast: Zucchini Bread Muffins
- Lunch: Eggplant Parmesan Stack
- Dinner: Sweet Potato and Black Bean Enchiladas
- Snack: Zucchini Fritters
- Dessert: Dark Chocolate Dipped Strawberries

Day 16

- Breakfast: Spinach and Mushroom Breakfast Burrito
- Lunch: Lentil and Vegetable Soup
- Dinner: Spaghetti Squash with Marinara Sauce
- Snack: Hummus with Carrot and Cucumber Sticks
- Dessert: Dark Chocolate Avocado Mousse

Day 17

- Breakfast: Greek Yogurt with Berries and Nuts
- Lunch: Chickpea and Avocado Salad
- Dinner: Baked Tofu with Steamed Vegetables
- Snack: Baked Kale Chips
- Dessert: Baked Apples with Cinnamon

Day 18

- Breakfast: Avocado Toast with Tomato and Basil
- Lunch: Quinoa and Black Bean Stuffed Peppers
- Dinner: Mushroom and Spinach Lasagna
- Snack: Roasted Chickpeas
- Dessert: Chia Seed Pudding with Mango

Day 19

- Breakfast: Chia Seed Pudding with Almond Milk
- Lunch: Grilled Vegetable Wrap
- Dinner: Stuffed Bell Peppers with Quinoa and Vegetables
- Snack: Edamame with Sea Salt
- Dessert: Berry and Greek Yogurt Parfait

Day 20

- Breakfast: Scrambled Tofu with Vegetables
- Lunch: Spinach and Feta Stuffed Portobellos

- Dinner: Vegetable and Bean Enchiladas
- Snack: Stuffed Mini Bell Peppers
- Dessert: Almond Flour Brownies

Day 21

- Breakfast: Overnight Oats with Flaxseeds
- Lunch: Zucchini Noodles with Pesto
- Dinner: Cauliflower Crust Pizza with Veggies
- Snack: Guacamole with Whole Grain Crackers
- Dessert: Banana and Oat Cookies

Week 4

Day 22

- Breakfast: Veggie-Packed Frittata
- Lunch: Roasted Beet and Arugula Salad
- Dinner: Lentil Shepherd's Pie
- Snack: Almond and Date Energy Balls
- Dessert: Coconut Flour Chocolate Cake

Day 23

- Breakfast: Quinoa Breakfast Bowl
- Lunch: Sweet Potato and Lentil Buddha Bowl
- Dinner: Eggplant Stir-Fry with Tofu

- Snack: Veggie Spring Rolls with Peanut Sauce
- Dessert: Mixed Berry Crumble

Day 24

- Breakfast: Smoothie Bowl with Fresh Fruits
- Lunch: Vegetable Stir-Fry with Brown Rice
- Dinner: Zucchini and Corn Tacos
- Snack: Greek Yogurt Dip with Veggies
- Dessert: Frozen Yogurt Bark with Berries

Day 25

- Breakfast: Whole Grain Pancakes with Berry Compote
- Lunch: Tomato Basil Soup with Whole Grain Bread
- Dinner: Vegetable Paella
- Snack: Caprese Salad Skewers
- Dessert: Apple Cinnamon Muffins

Day 26

- Breakfast: Sweet Potato and Black Bean Hash
- Lunch: Cauliflower Rice Burrito Bowl
- Dinner: Grilled Vegetable Skewers with Couscous
- Snack: Spicy Roasted Cauliflower Bites
- Dessert: Carrot Cake Energy Balls

Day 27

- Breakfast: Cottage Cheese with Pineapple and Walnuts
- Lunch: Mediterranean Chickpea Salad
- Dinner: Moroccan Chickpea Stew
- Snack: Avocado and Bean Dip
- Dessert: Peach Sorbet

Day 28

- Breakfast: Almond Butter Banana Sandwich
- Lunch: Tofu and Broccoli Salad with Peanut Dressing
- Dinner: Spinach and Ricotta Stuffed Shells
- Snack: Mini Quinoa Patties
- Dessert: Sugar-Free Lemon Bars

Day 29

- Breakfast: Berry and Spinach Smoothie
- Lunch: Mixed Bean Chili
- Dinner: Broccoli and Tofu Stir-Fry
- Snack: Apple Slices with Almond Butter
- Dessert: Pumpkin Spice Bites

Day 30

- Breakfast: Zucchini Bread Muffins
- Lunch: Eggplant Parmesan Stack

- Dinner: Sweet Potato and Black Bean Enchiladas
- Snack: Zucchini Fritters
- Dessert: Dark Chocolate Dipped Strawberries

Chapter 2: Breakfast Recipes

Starting your day with a nutritious and delicious breakfast is essential, especially for individuals managing type 2 diabetes. These breakfast recipes are designed to be quick, healthy, and packed with nutrients to keep you energized throughout the morning.

Spinach and Mushroom Breakfast Burrito

Ingredients:

- 1 whole wheat tortilla
- 1 cup fresh spinach
- 1/2 cup mushrooms, sliced
- 1/4 cup shredded low-fat cheese
- 2 eggs, beaten
- 1 tablespoon olive oil
- Salt and pepper to taste

Instructions:

1. Heat olive oil in a pan over medium heat.
2. Sauté mushrooms until soft, then add spinach and cook until wilted.
3. Pour in beaten eggs, stirring until scrambled and fully cooked.

4. Place the mixture onto the tortilla, sprinkle with cheese, and wrap.

Nutrition Information:

- Calories: 320
- Protein: 20g
- Carbohydrates: 28g
- Fat: 15g
- Fiber: 6g
- Sugar: 3g
- Portion Size: 1 burrito

Greek Yogurt with Berries and Nuts

Ingredients:

- 1 cup Greek yogurt
- 1/2 cup mixed berries (blueberries, strawberries, raspberries)
- 2 tablespoons mixed nuts (almonds, walnuts)
- 1 teaspoon honey (optional)

Instructions:

1. Place Greek yogurt in a bowl.
2. Top with mixed berries and nuts.
3. Drizzle with honey, if using.

Nutrition Information:

- Calories: 220
- Protein: 15g
- Carbohydrates: 18g
- Fat: 9g
- Fiber: 3g
- Sugar: 12g
- Portion Size: 1 bowl

Avocado Toast with Tomato and Basil

Ingredients:

- 1 slice whole grain bread
- 1/2 avocado, mashed
- 1 small tomato, sliced
- Fresh basil leaves
- Salt and pepper to taste

Instructions:

1. Toast the bread.
2. Spread mashed avocado on the toast.
3. Top with tomato slices and basil leaves.
4. Season with salt and pepper.

Nutrition Information:

- Calories: 210
- Protein: 4g
- Carbohydrates: 22g
- Fat: 12g
- Fiber: 7g
- Sugar: 3g
- Portion Size: 1 toast

Chia Seed Pudding with Almond Milk

Ingredients:

- 1/4 cup chia seeds
- 1 cup unsweetened almond milk
- 1 teaspoon vanilla extract
- 1 tablespoon maple syrup
- Fresh berries for topping

Instructions:

1. Mix chia seeds, almond milk, vanilla, and maple syrup in a bowl.
2. Refrigerate overnight.
3. Top with fresh berries before serving.

Nutrition Information:

- Calories: 250
- Protein: 6g
- Carbohydrates: 30g
- Fat: 12g
- Fiber: 10g
- Sugar: 10g
- Portion Size: 1 bowl

Scrambled Tofu with Vegetables

Ingredients:

- 1 block firm tofu, crumbled
- 1/2 cup bell peppers, diced
- 1/2 cup spinach
- 1 tablespoon olive oil
- 1 teaspoon turmeric
- Salt and pepper to taste

Instructions:

1. Heat olive oil in a pan over medium heat.
2. Add bell peppers and cook until soft.
3. Add crumbled tofu and turmeric, stirring well.
4. Add spinach and cook until wilted.

5. Season with salt and pepper.

Nutrition Information:

- Calories: 180
- Protein: 15g
- Carbohydrates: 8g
- Fat: 12g
- Fiber: 3g
- Sugar: 2g
- Portion Size: 1 serving

Overnight Oats with Flaxseeds

Ingredients:

- 1/2 cup rolled oats
- 1 cup unsweetened almond milk
- 1 tablespoon flaxseeds
- 1 teaspoon honey
- 1/2 cup blueberries

Instructions:

1. Combine oats, almond milk, flaxseeds, and honey in a jar.
2. Refrigerate overnight.
3. Top with blueberries before serving.

Nutrition Information:

- Calories: 220
- Protein: 6g
- Carbohydrates: 36g
- Fat: 6g
- Fiber: 8g
- Sugar: 10g
- Portion Size: 1 jar

Veggie-Packed Frittata

Ingredients:

- 6 eggs
- 1/2 cup cherry tomatoes, halved
- 1/2 cup spinach
- 1/4 cup onion, diced
- 1/4 cup bell peppers, diced
- 1/4 cup low-fat cheese, shredded
- 1 tablespoon olive oil
- Salt and pepper to taste

Instructions:

1. Preheat oven to 350°F (175°C).
2. Heat olive oil in an oven-safe skillet.

3. Sauté onions and bell peppers until soft.

4. Add tomatoes and spinach, cooking until spinach wilts.

5. Beat eggs and pour into the skillet, cooking until edges set.

6. Sprinkle cheese on top and transfer to the oven, baking until fully set.

Nutrition Information:

- Calories: 180
- Protein: 14g
- Carbohydrates: 5g
- Fat: 12g
- Fiber: 1g
- Sugar: 2g
- Portion Size: 1 slice

Quinoa Breakfast Bowl

Ingredients:

- 1/2 cup cooked quinoa
- 1/2 cup almond milk
- 1 tablespoon almond butter
- 1 teaspoon honey
- 1/2 cup sliced strawberries
- 1 tablespoon chia seeds

Instructions:

1. Warm quinoa and almond milk in a saucepan.

2. Stir in almond butter and honey.

3. Transfer to a bowl and top with strawberries and chia seeds.

Nutrition Information:

- Calories: 310
- Protein: 9g
- Carbohydrates: 45g
- Fat: 12g
- Fiber: 7g
- Sugar: 12g
- Portion Size: 1 bowl

Smoothie Bowl with Fresh Fruits

Ingredients:

- 1 banana, frozen
- 1/2 cup frozen berries
- 1/2 cup unsweetened almond milk
- 1 tablespoon chia seeds
- Fresh fruit and granola for topping

Instructions:

1. Blend banana, frozen berries, and almond milk until smooth.
2. Pour into a bowl and top with chia seeds, fresh fruit, and granola.

Nutrition Information:

- Calories: 250
- Protein: 5g
- Carbohydrates: 52g
- Fat: 6g
- Fiber: 10g
- Sugar: 26g
- Portion Size: 1 bowl

Whole Grain Pancakes with Berry Compote

Ingredients:

- 1 cup whole grain flour
- 1 tablespoon baking powder
- 1 cup almond milk
- 1 egg
- 1 tablespoon honey
- 1 cup mixed berries

- 1 tablespoon lemon juice

Instructions:

1. Mix flour and baking powder in a bowl.
2. Whisk almond milk, egg, and honey in another bowl, then combine with dry ingredients.
3. Cook pancakes on a griddle over medium heat.
4. For compote, heat berries and lemon juice in a saucepan until berries break down.

Nutrition Information:

- Calories: 320
- Protein: 9g
- Carbohydrates: 58g
- Fat: 8g
- Fiber: 10g
- Sugar: 20g
- Portion Size: 2 pancakes

Sweet Potato and Black Bean Hash

Ingredients:

- 1 sweet potato, diced
- 1/2 cup black beans, drained and rinsed

- 1/4 cup bell peppers, diced
- 1/4 cup onion, diced
- 1 tablespoon olive oil
- Salt and pepper to taste

Instructions:

1. Heat olive oil in a pan over medium heat.
2. Sauté onions and bell peppers until soft.
3. Add sweet potato and cook until tender.
4. Stir in black beans and season with salt and pepper.

Nutrition Information:

- Calories: 220
- Protein: 6g
- Carbohydrates: 38g
- Fat: 6g
- Fiber: 8g
- Sugar: 6g
- Portion Size: 1 bowl

Cottage Cheese with Pineapple and Walnuts

Ingredients:

- 1 cup cottage cheese
- 1/2 cup pineapple chunks
- 2 tablespoons walnuts, chopped

Instructions:

1. Place cottage cheese in a bowl.
2. Top with pineapple chunks and walnuts.

Nutrition Information:

- Calories: 200
- Protein: 15g
- Carbohydrates: 16g
- Fat: 9g
- Fiber: 2g
- Sugar: 10g
- Portion Size: 1 bowl

Almond Butter Banana Sandwich

Ingredients:

- 2 slices whole grain bread

- 2 tablespoons almond butter

- 1 banana, sliced

Instructions:

1. Spread almond butter on both slices of bread.

2. Layer banana slices on one slice and top with the other.

Nutrition Information:

- Calories: 340

- Protein: 10g

- Carbohydrates: 50g

- Fat: 14g

- Fiber: 8g

- Sugar: 14g

- Portion Size: 1 sandwich

Berry and Spinach Smoothie

Ingredients:

- 1 cup spinach

- 1/2 cup mixed berries

- 1 banana

- 1 cup almond milk

Instructions:

1. Blend spinach, berries, banana, and almond milk until smooth.

Nutrition Information:

- Calories: 180
- Protein: 3g
- Carbohydrates: 36g
- Fat: 3g
- Fiber: 6g
- Sugar: 20g
- Portion Size: 1 smoothie

Zucchini Bread Muffins

Ingredients:

- 1 cup whole wheat flour
- 1/2 cup almond flour
- 1 teaspoon baking powder
- 1 teaspoon baking soda
- 1 teaspoon cinnamon
- 1 cup grated zucchini
- 1/2 cup unsweetened applesauce
- 1/4 cup honey

- 1 egg
- 1 teaspoon vanilla extract

Instructions:

1. Preheat oven to 350°F (175°C).
2. Mix dry ingredients in one bowl.
3. Combine wet ingredients and zucchini in another bowl.
4. Combine both mixtures and pour into muffin tins.
5. Bake for 20-25 minutes.

Nutrition Information:

- Calories: 120
- Protein: 3g
- Carbohydrates: 20g
- Fat: 4g
- Fiber: 3g
- Sugar: 10g
- Portion Size: 1 muffin

Chapter 3: Lunch Recipes

Eating a balanced and nutritious lunch is essential to maintaining energy levels and supporting overall health throughout the day. This chapter presents a variety of delicious and wholesome lunch recipes that cater to diverse tastes and dietary preferences.

Lentil and Vegetable Soup

Ingredients:

- 1 cup green lentils, rinsed
- 1 onion, chopped
- 2 carrots, chopped
- 2 celery stalks, chopped
- 3 garlic cloves, minced
- 1 can (14.5 oz) diced tomatoes
- 6 cups vegetable broth
- 1 tsp dried thyme
- 1 tsp cumin
- Salt and pepper to taste

Instructions:

1. In a large pot, sauté onion, carrots, and celery until tender.
2. Add garlic and cook for another minute.

3. Stir in lentils, tomatoes, broth, thyme, and cumin.

4. Bring to a boil, then reduce heat and simmer for 30 minutes.

5. Season with salt and pepper.

Nutrition Information:

- Calories: 220
- Protein: 12g
- Carbohydrates: 35g
- Fat: 2g
- Fiber: 12g
- Sugar: 7g
- Portion Size: 1 cup

Chickpea and Avocado Salad

Ingredients:

- 1 can (15 oz) chickpeas, rinsed and drained
- 1 avocado, diced
- 1 cucumber, diced
- 1 bell pepper, diced
- 1/4 red onion, finely chopped
- 2 tbsp olive oil
- 1 tbsp lemon juice
- Salt and pepper to taste

Instructions:

1. In a bowl, combine chickpeas, avocado, cucumber, bell pepper, and red onion.
2. Drizzle with olive oil and lemon juice.
3. Toss gently to combine.
4. Season with salt and pepper.

Nutrition Information:

- Calories: 280
- Protein: 6g
- Carbohydrates: 27g
- Fat: 18g
- Fiber: 10g
- Sugar: 3g
- Portion Size: 1 cup

Quinoa and Black Bean Stuffed Peppers

Ingredients:

- 4 bell peppers, halved and seeds removed
- 1 cup cooked quinoa
- 1 can (15 oz) black beans, rinsed and drained
- 1 cup corn kernels
- 1 tsp cumin

- 1 tsp chili powder
- 1/2 cup salsa
- Salt and pepper to taste

Instructions:

1. Preheat oven to 375°F (190°C).
2. In a bowl, mix quinoa, black beans, corn, cumin, chili powder, and salsa.
3. Stuff the bell peppers with the mixture.
4. Place peppers in a baking dish and bake for 25-30 minutes.

Nutrition Information:

- Calories: 250
- Protein: 10g
- Carbohydrates: 45g
- Fat: 4g
- Fiber: 12g
- Sugar: 7g
- Portion Size: 1 stuffed pepper half

Grilled Vegetable Wrap

Ingredients:

- 1 zucchini, sliced

- 1 red bell pepper, sliced
- 1 yellow bell pepper, sliced
- 1 red onion, sliced
- 2 tbsp olive oil
- Salt and pepper to taste
- 4 whole wheat tortillas
- 1/2 cup hummus
- 1 cup mixed greens

Instructions:

1. Toss vegetables with olive oil, salt, and pepper.
2. Grill vegetables until tender and slightly charred.
3. Spread hummus on each tortilla.
4. Add grilled vegetables and mixed greens.
5. Roll up and slice in half.

Nutrition Information:

- Calories: 320
- Protein: 8g
- Carbohydrates: 42g
- Fat: 14g
- Fiber: 8g
- Sugar: 6g
- Portion Size: 1 wrap

Spinach and Feta Stuffed Portobellos

Ingredients:

- 4 large portobello mushrooms, stems removed
- 1 cup spinach, chopped
- 1/2 cup feta cheese, crumbled
- 1 garlic clove, minced
- 1 tbsp olive oil
- Salt and pepper to taste

Instructions:

1. Preheat oven to 375°F (190°C).
2. Sauté spinach and garlic in olive oil until wilted.
3. Mix spinach with feta cheese.
4. Stuff mushrooms with the mixture.
5. Bake for 20 minutes.

Nutrition Information:

- Calories: 180
- Protein: 8g
- Carbohydrates: 10g
- Fat: 14g
- Fiber: 3g
- Sugar: 3g
- Portion Size: 1 stuffed mushroom

Zucchini Noodles with Pesto

Ingredients:

- 4 zucchinis, spiralized
- 1/2 cup basil pesto
- 1/4 cup cherry tomatoes, halved
- 2 tbsp pine nuts, toasted
- Salt and pepper to taste

Instructions:

1. Toss zucchini noodles with pesto.
2. Add cherry tomatoes and pine nuts.
3. Season with salt and pepper.

Nutrition Information:

- Calories: 250
- Protein: 6g
- Carbohydrates: 15g
- Fat: 20g
- Fiber: 4g
- Sugar: 7g
- Portion Size: 1 cup

Roasted Beet and Arugula Salad

Ingredients:

- 4 beets, roasted and sliced
- 4 cups arugula
- 1/4 red onion, thinly sliced
- 1/4 cup goat cheese, crumbled
- 2 tbsp balsamic vinegar
- 2 tbsp olive oil
- Salt and pepper to taste

Instructions:

1. Arrange arugula on a plate.
2. Top with roasted beets, red onion, and goat cheese.
3. Drizzle with balsamic vinegar and olive oil.
4. Season with salt and pepper.

Nutrition Information:

- Calories: 220
- Protein: 6g
- Carbohydrates: 24g
- Fat: 12g
- Fiber: 6g
- Sugar: 15g
- Portion Size: 1 cup

Sweet Potato and Lentil Buddha Bowl

Ingredients:

- 2 sweet potatoes, roasted and diced
- 1 cup cooked lentils
- 2 cups mixed greens
- 1/2 avocado, sliced
- 1/4 cup tahini dressing

Instructions:

1. Arrange sweet potatoes, lentils, and mixed greens in a bowl.
2. Top with avocado slices.
3. Drizzle with tahini dressing.

Nutrition Information:

- Calories: 350
- Protein: 12g
- Carbohydrates: 50g
- Fat: 14g
- Fiber: 14g
- Sugar: 8g
- Portion Size: 1 bowl

Vegetable Stir-Fry with Brown Rice

Ingredients:

- 2 cups mixed vegetables (broccoli, bell peppers, carrots)
- 1 cup cooked brown rice
- 2 tbsp soy sauce
- 1 tbsp sesame oil
- 1 garlic clove, minced
- 1 tsp ginger, grated

Instructions:

1. Sauté garlic and ginger in sesame oil.
2. Add mixed vegetables and stir-fry until tender.
3. Stir in cooked brown rice and soy sauce.

Nutrition Information:

- Calories: 300
- Protein: 8g
- Carbohydrates: 50g
- Fat: 8g
- Fiber: 6g
- Sugar: 4g
- Portion Size: 1 cup

Tomato Basil Soup with Whole Grain Bread

Ingredients:

- 2 tbsp olive oil
- 1 onion, chopped
- 3 garlic cloves, minced
- 6 cups tomatoes, chopped
- 2 cups vegetable broth
- 1/2 cup fresh basil, chopped
- Salt and pepper to taste
- Whole grain bread for serving

Instructions:

1. Sauté onion and garlic in olive oil.
2. Add tomatoes and broth, and simmer for 20 minutes.
3. Blend until smooth and stir in basil.
4. Season with salt and pepper.
5. Serve with whole grain bread.

Nutrition Information:

- Calories: 180
- Protein: 6g
- Carbohydrates: 30g
- Fat: 6g

- Fiber: 4g

- Sugar: 12g

- Portion Size: 1 cup soup with 1 slice bread

Cauliflower Rice Burrito Bowl

Ingredients:

- 1 head cauliflower, riced

- 1 cup black beans, rinsed and drained

- 1 cup corn kernels

- 1 avocado, diced

- 1/4 cup salsa

- 1 lime, juiced

- Salt and pepper to taste

Instructions:

1. Sauté cauliflower rice in a pan until tender.

2. Arrange cauliflower rice, black beans, corn, and avocado in a bowl.

3. Top with salsa and lime juice.

4. Season with salt and pepper.

Nutrition Information:

- Calories: 280

- Protein: 10g

- Carbohydrates: 36g

- Fat: 12g

- Fiber: 12g

- Sugar: 6g

- Portion Size: 1 bowl

Mediterranean Chickpea Salad

Ingredients:

- 1 can (15 oz) chickpeas, rinsed and drained

- 1/2 cucumber, diced

- 1/2 red bell pepper, diced

- 1/4 red onion, finely chopped

- 1/4 cup feta cheese, crumbled

- 2 tbsp olive oil

- 1 tbsp lemon juice

- 1 tsp dried oregano

- Salt and pepper to taste

Instructions:

1. In a bowl, combine chickpeas, cucumber, bell pepper, red onion, and feta cheese.

2. Drizzle with olive oil and lemon juice.

3. Sprinkle with oregano.

4. Season with salt and pepper.

Nutrition Information:

- Calories: 240

- Protein: 8g

- Carbohydrates: 30g

- Fat: 10g

- Fiber: 8g

- Sugar: 5g

- Portion Size: 1 cup

Tofu and Broccoli Salad with Peanut Dressing

Ingredients:

- 1 block firm tofu, cubed

- 2 cups broccoli florets

- 1/4 cup peanut butter

- 2 tbsp soy sauce

- 1 tbsp lime juice

- 1 tbsp honey

- 1 garlic clove, minced

- 1 tsp ginger, grated

Instructions:

1. Steam broccoli until tender.

2. Mix peanut butter, soy sauce, lime juice, honey, garlic, and ginger to make the dressing.

3. Combine tofu and broccoli in a bowl.

4. Toss with peanut dressing.

Nutrition Information:

- Calories: 320
- Protein: 18g
- Carbohydrates: 20g
- Fat: 20g
- Fiber: 6g
- Sugar: 8g
- Portion Size: 1 bowl

Mixed Bean Chili

Ingredients:

- 1 can (15 oz) kidney beans, rinsed and drained
- 1 can (15 oz) black beans, rinsed and drained
- 1 can (15 oz) pinto beans, rinsed and drained
- 1 onion, chopped
- 2 garlic cloves, minced

- 1 can (14.5 oz) diced tomatoes

- 2 cups vegetable broth

- 1 tbsp chili powder

- 1 tsp cumin

- Salt and pepper to taste

Instructions:

1. Sauté onion and garlic until tender.

2. Add beans, tomatoes, broth, chili powder, and cumin.

3. Simmer for 30 minutes.

4. Season with salt and pepper.

Nutrition Information:

- Calories: 280

- Protein: 14g

- Carbohydrates: 45g

- Fat: 4g

- Fiber: 15g

- Sugar: 6g

- Portion Size: 1 cup

Eggplant Parmesan Stack

Ingredients:

- 1 large eggplant, sliced
- 1 cup marinara sauce
- 1 cup mozzarella cheese, shredded
- 1/4 cup Parmesan cheese, grated
- 1/4 cup fresh basil, chopped
- 2 tbsp olive oil
- Salt and pepper to taste

Instructions:

1. Preheat oven to 375°F (190°C).
2. Brush eggplant slices with olive oil and season with salt and pepper.
3. Roast eggplant for 20 minutes.
4. Layer eggplant slices with marinara sauce and cheeses.
5. Bake for another 15 minutes.
6. Garnish with fresh basil.

Nutrition Information:

- Calories: 320
- Protein: 12g
- Carbohydrates: 20g
- Fat: 22g

- Fiber: 8g
- Sugar: 10g
- Portion Size: 1 stack

Chapter 4: Dinner Recipes

In this Chapter, you'll discover a variety of satisfying dinner options that are both nutritious and flavorful. From hearty casseroles to savory stir-fries, these recipes are designed to keep you feeling satisfied and energized. Each recipe is carefully crafted with wholesome ingredients to support your health goals.

Spaghetti Squash with Marinara Sauce

Ingredients:

- 1 medium spaghetti squash
- 2 cups marinara sauce
- Salt and pepper to taste
- Fresh basil for garnish

Instructions:

1. Preheat oven to 400°F (200°C).
2. Cut spaghetti squash in half lengthwise and remove seeds.
3. Place squash halves cut-side down on a baking sheet and bake for 30-40 minutes, until tender.
4. Scrape the flesh of the squash with a fork to create "spaghetti" strands.
5. Heat marinara sauce in a saucepan over medium heat.

6. Serve spaghetti squash topped with marinara sauce and garnish with fresh basil.

Nutrition Information (per serving):

- Calories: 180
- Protein: 4g
- Carbohydrates: 40g
- Fat: 2g
- Fiber: 10g
- Sugar: 15g
- Portion Size: 1/2 squash with sauce

Baked Tofu with Steamed Vegetables

Ingredients:

- 1 block extra firm tofu, pressed and cubed
- 2 cups mixed vegetables (such as broccoli, carrots, and bell peppers)
- 2 tablespoons soy sauce
- 1 tablespoon olive oil
- Salt and pepper to taste

Instructions:

1. Preheat oven to 400°F (200°C).

2. Arrange tofu cubes on a baking sheet lined with parchment paper.

3. Drizzle tofu with soy sauce and olive oil, then season with salt and pepper.

4. Bake tofu for 25-30 minutes, until golden brown and crispy.

5. Steam mixed vegetables until tender.

6. Serve baked tofu with steamed vegetables.

Nutrition Information (per serving):

- Calories: 220
- Protein: 15g
- Carbohydrates: 15g
- Fat: 12g
- Fiber: 5g
- Sugar: 5g
- Portion Size: 1/4 tofu with vegetables

Mushroom and Spinach Lasagna

Ingredients:

- 9 lasagna noodles
- 2 cups marinara sauce
- 2 cups sliced mushrooms
- 2 cups fresh spinach

- 1 cup ricotta cheese
- 1 cup shredded mozzarella cheese
- Salt and pepper to taste

Instructions:

1. Preheat oven to 375°F (190°C).
2. Cook lasagna noodles according to package instructions, then drain and set aside.
3. In a skillet, sauté mushrooms until golden brown.
4. In a separate bowl, mix together ricotta cheese, spinach, salt, and pepper.
5. Spread a thin layer of marinara sauce on the bottom of a baking dish.
6. Layer noodles, mushroom mixture, spinach mixture, and mozzarella cheese in the baking dish.
7. Repeat layers until ingredients are used up, ending with a layer of cheese on top.
8. Cover with foil and bake for 25 minutes, then uncover and bake for an additional 10 minutes until cheese is bubbly.
9. Let lasagna cool for a few minutes before serving.

Nutrition Information (per serving):

- Calories: 320
- Protein: 20g

- Carbohydrates: 30g

- Fat: 15g

- Fiber: 5g

- Sugar: 8g

- Portion Size: 1/6 lasagna

Stuffed Bell Peppers with Quinoa and Vegetables

Ingredients:

- 4 large bell peppers, halved and seeds removed

- 1 cup cooked quinoa

- 1 cup black beans, drained and rinsed

- 1 cup corn kernels

- 1 cup diced tomatoes

- 1/2 cup diced onion

- 1/2 cup shredded cheddar cheese

- 1 teaspoon chili powder

- Salt and pepper to taste

Instructions:

1. Preheat oven to 375°F (190°C).

2. In a large bowl, mix together cooked quinoa, black beans, corn, diced tomatoes, onion, chili powder, salt, and pepper.

3. Stuff each bell pepper half with the quinoa mixture.

4. Place stuffed peppers in a baking dish and cover with foil.

5. Bake for 25 minutes, then remove foil and sprinkle shredded cheese on top of each pepper.

6. Bake for an additional 10 minutes until cheese is melted and peppers are tender.

7. Serve hot.

Nutrition Information (per serving):

- Calories: 250
- Protein: 12g
- Carbohydrates: 35g
- Fat: 8g
- Fiber: 8g
- Sugar: 10g
- Portion Size: 1/2 stuffed pepper

Vegetable and Bean Enchiladas

Ingredients:

- 8 whole wheat tortillas
- 2 cups cooked black beans
- 2 cups mixed vegetables (such as bell peppers, onions, and zucchini)

- 1 cup enchilada sauce

- 1 cup shredded cheddar cheese

- 1/2 cup chopped cilantro

- Salt and pepper to taste

Instructions:

1. Preheat oven to 375°F (190°C).

2. In a skillet, sauté mixed vegetables until tender.

3. Warm tortillas in the microwave or on a skillet.

4. Spread a spoonful of enchilada sauce on each tortilla.

5. Fill tortillas with cooked black beans and sautéed vegetables.

6. Roll up tortillas and place seam-side down in a baking dish.

7. Pour remaining enchilada sauce over the rolled tortillas.

8. Sprinkle shredded cheese on top of enchiladas.

9. Bake for 20 minutes, until cheese is melted and bubbly.

10. Garnish with chopped cilantro before serving.

Nutrition Information (per serving):

- Calories: 320

- Protein: 15g

- Carbohydrates: 40g

- Fat: 12g

- Fiber: 8g

- Sugar: 5g

- Portion Size: 2 enchiladas

Cauliflower Crust Pizza with Veggies

Ingredients:

- 1 cauliflower head, grated
- 2 eggs
- 1/2 cup shredded mozzarella cheese
- 1 teaspoon Italian seasoning
- 1 cup marinara sauce
- 1 cup mixed vegetables (such as bell peppers, mushrooms, and onions)
- 1/2 cup shredded Parmesan cheese
- Salt and pepper to taste

Instructions:

1. Preheat oven to 425°F (220°C).
2. Mix grated cauliflower, eggs, mozzarella cheese, Italian seasoning, salt, and pepper in a bowl.
3. Press cauliflower mixture onto a parchment-lined baking sheet to form a pizza crust.
4. Bake crust for 20 minutes, until golden brown and firm.
5. Spread marinara sauce over the baked crust.
6. Top with mixed vegetables and shredded Parmesan cheese.

7. Bake for an additional 10-15 minutes, until cheese is melted and bubbly.

8. Slice and serve hot.

Nutrition Information (per serving):

- Calories: 180
- Protein: 10g
- Carbohydrates: 20g
- Fat: 8g
- Fiber: 6g
- Sugar: 8g
- Portion Size: 1/4 pizza

Lentil Shepherd's Pie

Ingredients:

- 2 cups cooked lentils
- 2 cups mashed potatoes
- 1 cup diced carrots
- 1 cup frozen peas
- 1 cup diced onion
- 2 cloves garlic, minced
- 1 cup vegetable broth
- 2 tablespoons tomato paste

- 1 tablespoon olive oil
- Salt and pepper to taste

Instructions:

1. Preheat oven to 375°F (190°C).
2. In a skillet, sauté diced onion and minced garlic in olive oil until softened.
3. Add diced carrots, frozen peas, cooked lentils, vegetable broth, tomato paste, salt, and pepper to the skillet.
4. Cook until vegetables are tender and mixture is thickened.
5. Transfer lentil mixture to a baking dish and spread mashed potatoes over the top.
6. Bake for 25 minutes, until mashed potatoes are golden brown.
7. Serve hot.

Nutrition Information (per serving):

- Calories: 280
- Protein: 12g
- Carbohydrates: 40g
- Fat: 8g
- Fiber: 10g
- Sugar: 8g
- Portion Size: 1/6 pie

Eggplant Stir-Fry with Tofu

Ingredients:

- 1 large eggplant, diced
- 1 block firm tofu, cubed
- 2 cups mixed bell peppers, sliced
- 1 cup sliced mushrooms
- 1/4 cup soy sauce
- 2 tablespoons sesame oil
- 2 cloves garlic, minced
- 1 tablespoon ginger, grated
- 2 green onions, chopped
- Salt and pepper to taste

Instructions:

1. Press cubed tofu to remove excess moisture.
2. Heat sesame oil in a large skillet over medium heat.
3. Add minced garlic and grated ginger to the skillet and sauté for 1-2 minutes.
4. Add diced eggplant and cook until softened, about 5-7 minutes.
5. Add sliced bell peppers and mushrooms to the skillet and cook until tender.
6. Push vegetables to the side of the skillet and add cubed tofu.
7. Cook tofu until golden brown on all sides.

8. Stir in soy sauce and green onions, and season with salt and pepper.

9. Serve hot over cooked rice or quinoa.

Nutrition Information (per serving):

- Calories: 280

- Protein: 15g

- Carbohydrates: 20g

- Fat: 15g

- Fiber: 8g

- Sugar: 8g

- Portion Size: 1/4 stir-fry

Zucchini and Corn Tacos

Ingredients:

- 8 small corn tortillas

- 2 cups diced zucchini

- 1 cup corn kernels

- 1 cup black beans, drained and rinsed

- 1/2 cup diced onion

- 1/4 cup chopped cilantro

- 1 avocado, sliced

- 1 lime, cut into wedges

- Salt and pepper to taste

Instructions:

1. Warm corn tortillas in a skillet or microwave.
2. In a separate skillet, sauté diced zucchini and diced onion until tender.
3. Add corn kernels and black beans to the skillet and cook until heated through.
4. Season mixture with salt, pepper, and chopped cilantro.
5. Fill each tortilla with the zucchini and corn mixture.
6. Top with sliced avocado and a squeeze of lime juice.
7. Serve hot.

Nutrition Information (per serving):

- Calories: 220
- Protein: 8g
- Carbohydrates: 30g
- Fat: 10g
- Fiber: 10g
- Sugar: 5g
- Portion Size: 2 tacos

Vegetable Paella

Ingredients:

- 1 cup Arborio rice
- 2 cups vegetable broth
- 1 cup diced tomatoes
- 1 cup mixed vegetables (such as bell peppers, peas, and carrots)
- 1/2 cup diced onion
- 2 cloves garlic, minced
- 1 teaspoon smoked paprika
- 1/2 teaspoon saffron threads
- 1/4 cup chopped parsley
- Salt and pepper to taste
- Lemon wedges for serving

Instructions:

1. In a large skillet, sauté diced onion and minced garlic until translucent.
2. Add Arborio rice to the skillet and cook for 2-3 minutes, stirring constantly.
3. Stir in diced tomatoes, mixed vegetables, smoked paprika, saffron threads, salt, and pepper.
4. Pour vegetable broth into the skillet and bring to a simmer.

5. Cover and cook for 20-25 minutes, until rice is tender and liquid is absorbed.

6. Fluff rice with a fork and sprinkle chopped parsley on top.

7. Serve hot with lemon wedges on the side.

Nutrition Information (per serving):

- Calories: 250

- Protein: 6g

- Carbohydrates: 50g

- Fat: 2g

- Fiber: 5g

- Sugar: 5g

- Portion Size: 1/4 paella

Grilled Vegetable Skewers with Couscous

Ingredients:

- 1 zucchini, sliced

- 1 yellow squash, sliced

- 1 red bell pepper, diced

- 1 yellow bell pepper, diced

- 1 red onion, diced

- 1 cup cherry tomatoes

- 1 cup cooked couscous
- 2 tablespoons olive oil
- 1 tablespoon balsamic vinegar
- 1 teaspoon Italian seasoning
- Salt and pepper to taste

Instructions:

1. Preheat grill to medium-high heat.
2. Thread sliced vegetables onto skewers, alternating colors.
3. In a small bowl, whisk together olive oil, balsamic vinegar, Italian seasoning, salt, and pepper.
4. Brush vegetable skewers with the olive oil mixture.
5. Grill skewers for 10-12 minutes, turning occasionally, until vegetables are tender and slightly charred.
6. Serve grilled vegetable skewers over cooked couscous.

Nutrition Information (per serving):

- Calories: 220
- Protein: 6g
- Carbohydrates: 40g
- Fat: 6g
- Fiber: 8g
- Sugar: 8g
- Portion Size: 2 skewers with couscous

Moroccan Chickpea Stew

Ingredients:

- 2 cups cooked chickpeas
- 1 onion, chopped
- 2 cloves garlic, minced
- 1 bell pepper, diced
- 1 carrot, diced
- 1 zucchini, diced
- 1 cup diced tomatoes
- 3 cups vegetable broth
- 1 teaspoon ground cumin
- 1 teaspoon ground coriander
- 1/2 teaspoon ground cinnamon
- 1/4 teaspoon cayenne pepper
- Salt and pepper to taste
- Fresh cilantro for garnish

Instructions:

1. In a large pot, sauté chopped onion and minced garlic until fragrant.
2. Add diced bell pepper, carrot, and zucchini to the pot and cook until slightly softened.

3. Stir in diced tomatoes, cooked chickpeas, vegetable broth, ground cumin, ground coriander, ground cinnamon, cayenne pepper, salt, and pepper.

4. Bring stew to a simmer and cook for 20-25 minutes, until vegetables are tender and flavors are well combined.

5. Adjust seasoning to taste.

6. Serve hot, garnished with fresh cilantro.

Nutrition Information (per serving):

- Calories: 280
- Protein: 10g
- Carbohydrates: 45g
- Fat: 6g
- Fiber: 12g
- Sugar: 10g
- Portion Size: 1 1/2 cups stew

Spinach and Ricotta Stuffed Shells

Ingredients:

- 20 jumbo pasta shells
- 2 cups ricotta cheese
- 1 cup chopped spinach
- 1/2 cup grated Parmesan cheese

- 1 egg

- 2 cups marinara sauce

- 1 cup shredded mozzarella cheese

- Salt and pepper to taste

Instructions:

1. Preheat oven to 375°F (190°C).

2. Cook jumbo pasta shells according to package instructions, then drain and set aside.

3. In a bowl, mix together ricotta cheese, chopped spinach, grated Parmesan cheese, egg, salt, and pepper.

4. Spread a thin layer of marinara sauce on the bottom of a baking dish.

5. Stuff each cooked pasta shell with the ricotta mixture and place in the baking dish.

6. Pour remaining marinara sauce over the stuffed shells.

7. Sprinkle shredded mozzarella cheese on top.

8. Cover with foil and bake for 25 minutes.

9. Remove foil and bake for an additional 10 minutes, until cheese is melted and bubbly.

10. Serve hot.

Nutrition Information (per serving):

- Calories: 320

- Protein: 18g
- Carbohydrates: 35g
- Fat: 12g
- Fiber: 5g
- Sugar: 8g
- Portion Size: 5 stuffed shells

Broccoli and Tofu Stir-Fry

Ingredients:

- 1 block firm tofu, cubed
- 4 cups broccoli florets
- 1 bell pepper, sliced
- 1 carrot, julienned
- 1/2 cup sliced mushrooms
- 2 cloves garlic, minced
- 2 tablespoons soy sauce
- 1 tablespoon sesame oil
- 1 tablespoon rice vinegar
- 1 teaspoon cornstarch
- 1/4 cup vegetable broth
- Salt and pepper to taste
- Sesame seeds for garnish

Instructions:

1. Press cubed tofu to remove excess moisture.
2. Heat sesame oil in a large skillet over medium heat.
3. Add minced garlic to the skillet and sauté for 1-2 minutes.
4. Add cubed tofu to the skillet and cook until golden brown on all sides.
5. In a small bowl, whisk together soy sauce, rice vinegar, cornstarch, vegetable broth, salt, and pepper.
6. Add broccoli florets, sliced bell pepper, julienned carrot, and sliced mushrooms to the skillet.
7. Pour the sauce mixture over the tofu and vegetables.
8. Cook for 5-7 minutes, until vegetables are tender and sauce is thickened.
9. Serve hot, garnished with sesame seeds.

Nutrition Information (per serving):

- Calories: 250
- Protein: 15g
- Carbohydrates: 20g
- Fat: 12g
- Fiber: 8g
- Sugar: 5g
- Portion Size: 1/4 stir-fry

Sweet Potato and Black Bean Enchiladas

Ingredients:

- 8 small whole wheat tortillas
- 2 cups mashed sweet potato
- 1 cup cooked black beans
- 1 cup diced bell pepper
- 1/2 cup diced onion
- 1 cup enchilada sauce
- 1 cup shredded Monterey Jack cheese
- 1/4 cup chopped cilantro
- Salt and pepper to taste

Instructions:

1. Preheat oven to 375°F (190°C).
2. In a bowl, mix together mashed sweet potato, cooked black beans, diced bell pepper, diced onion, salt, and pepper.
3. Warm whole wheat tortillas in the microwave or on a skillet.
4. Spread a spoonful of enchilada sauce on each tortilla.
5. Fill tortillas with the sweet potato and black bean mixture.
6. Roll up tortillas and place seam-side down in a baking dish.
7. Pour remaining enchilada sauce over the rolled tortillas.
8. Sprinkle shredded cheese on top of enchiladas.
9. Bake for 20 minutes, until cheese is melted and bubbly.
10. Garnish with chopped cilantro before serving.

Nutrition Information (per serving):

- Calories: 320
- Protein: 15g
- Carbohydrates: 40g
- Fat: 12g
- Fiber: 8g
- Sugar: 5g
- Portion Size: 2 enchiladas

Chapter 5: Snacks and Appetizers

In this chapter, you'll find a collection of snacks and appetizers that are not only delicious but also packed with nutrients to keep you feeling satisfied and energized. Enjoy these recipes guilt-free knowing they're not only tasty but also good for you!

Hummus with Carrot and Cucumber Sticks

Ingredients:

- 1 cup of chickpeas
- 2 tablespoons of tahini
- 2 cloves of garlic
- Juice of 1 lemon
- 2 tablespoons of olive oil
- Salt and pepper to taste
- Carrot and cucumber sticks for dipping

Instructions:

1. In a food processor, combine chickpeas, tahini, garlic, lemon juice, olive oil, salt, and pepper.
2. Blend until smooth and creamy, adding water as needed to reach desired consistency.

3. Serve hummus with carrot and cucumber sticks for dipping.

Nutrition Information:

- Calories: 120
- Protein: 5g
- Carbohydrates: 10g
- Fat: 7g
- Fiber: 3g
- Sugar: 2g
- Portion Size: 2 tablespoons of hummus with 1 cup of veggies

Baked Kale Chips

Ingredients:

- 1 bunch of kale
- 1 tablespoon of olive oil
- Salt and pepper to taste

Instructions:

1. Preheat oven to 350°F (175°C).
2. Remove kale leaves from stems and tear into bite-sized pieces.
3. Drizzle kale with olive oil and sprinkle with salt and pepper.
4. Spread kale in a single layer on a baking sheet.

5. Bake for 10-15 minutes until crispy.

6. Allow to cool before serving.

Nutrition Information:

- Calories: 50

- Protein: 2g

- Carbohydrates: 5g

- Fat: 3g

- Fiber: 2g

- Sugar: 0g

- Portion Size: 1 cup of kale chips

Roasted Chickpeas

Ingredients:

- 1 can of chickpeas, drained and rinsed

- 1 tablespoon of olive oil

- 1 teaspoon of cumin

- 1 teaspoon of paprika

- Salt to taste

Instructions:

1. Preheat oven to 400°F (200°C).

2. Pat chickpeas dry with a paper towel.

3. In a bowl, toss chickpeas with olive oil, cumin, paprika, and salt.

4. Spread chickpeas in a single layer on a baking sheet.

5. Roast for 25-30 minutes until crispy, shaking the pan halfway through.

6. Allow to cool before serving.

Nutrition Information:

- Calories: 120
- Protein: 5g
- Carbohydrates: 15g
- Fat: 4g
- Fiber: 5g
- Sugar: 3g
- Portion Size: 1/4 cup of roasted chickpeas

Edamame with Sea Salt

Ingredients:

- 1 cup of edamame (shelled)
- Sea salt to taste

Instructions:

1. Boil a pot of water and add the edamame.

2. Cook for 3-5 minutes until tender.

3. Drain and sprinkle with sea salt.

4. Serve warm or chilled.

Nutrition Information:

- Calories: 120
- Protein: 11g
- Carbohydrates: 10g
- Fat: 3g
- Fiber: 5g
- Sugar: 3g
- Portion Size: 1 cup of edamame

Stuffed Mini Bell Peppers

Ingredients:

- 12 mini bell peppers
- 1 cup of cream cheese
- 1/4 cup of chopped fresh herbs (such as parsley, chives, or dill)
- Salt and pepper to taste

Instructions:

1. Cut the tops off the mini bell peppers and remove the seeds.

2. In a bowl, mix cream cheese, chopped herbs, salt, and pepper.

3. Stuff each pepper with the cream cheese mixture.

4. Serve chilled or at room temperature.

Nutrition Information:

- Calories: 60

- Protein: 2g

- Carbohydrates: 3g

- Fat: 5g

- Fiber: 1g

- Sugar: 2g

- Portion Size: 2 stuffed mini bell peppers

Guacamole with Whole Grain Crackers

Ingredients:

- 2 ripe avocados

- 1 tomato, diced

- 1/4 cup of diced red onion

- Juice of 1 lime

- Salt and pepper to taste

- Whole grain crackers for serving

Instructions:

1. Mash avocados in a bowl until smooth.
2. Stir in diced tomato, red onion, lime juice, salt, and pepper.
3. Serve guacamole with whole grain crackers.

Nutrition Information:

- Calories: 150
- Protein: 2g
- Carbohydrates: 10g
- Fat: 12g
- Fiber: 7g
- Sugar: 2g
- Portion Size: 1/4 cup of guacamole with 5 crackers

Almond and Date Energy Balls

Ingredients:

- 1 cup of almonds
- 1 cup of pitted dates
- 1 tablespoon of cocoa powder
- 1 tablespoon of almond butter
- Shredded coconut (optional, for rolling)

Instructions:

1. In a food processor, blend almonds until finely ground.
2. Add dates, cocoa powder, and almond butter. Blend until mixture sticks together.
3. Roll mixture into small balls.
4. Optional: Roll balls in shredded coconut.
5. Chill in the refrigerator before serving.

Nutrition Information:

- Calories: 80
- Protein: 2g
- Carbohydrates: 10g
- Fat: 4g
- Fiber: 2g
- Sugar: 7g
- Portion Size: 1 energy ball

Veggie Spring Rolls with Peanut Sauce

Ingredients:

- Rice paper wrappers
- Assorted vegetables (such as carrots, cucumbers, bell peppers, lettuce)
- Fresh herbs (such as cilantro, mint, basil)

- Peanut sauce for dipping

Instructions:

1. Prepare vegetables by slicing them into thin strips.
2. Dip a rice paper wrapper in warm water for a few seconds until softened.
3. Lay wrapper flat and place vegetables and herbs in the center.
4. Fold the sides of the wrapper over the filling, then roll tightly.
5. Serve with peanut sauce for dipping.

Nutrition Information:

- Calories: 70
- Protein: 2g
- Carbohydrates: 15g
- Fat: 1g
- Fiber: 3g
- Sugar: 2g
- Portion Size: 1 spring roll with 2 tablespoons of peanut sauce

Greek Yogurt Dip with Veggies

Ingredients:

- 1 cup of Greek yogurt
- 1 tablespoon of lemon juice
- 1 tablespoon of chopped fresh dill
- Salt and pepper to taste
- Assorted vegetables for dipping (such as carrots, cucumbers, bell peppers)

Instructions:

1. In a bowl, mix Greek yogurt, lemon juice, dill, salt, and pepper.
2. Serve with assorted vegetables for dipping.

Nutrition Information:

- Calories: 60
- Protein: 8g
- Carbohydrates: 5g
- Fat: 1g
- Fiber: 1g
- Sugar: 3g
- Portion Size: 1/4 cup of dip with 1 cup of veggies

Caprese Salad Skewers

Ingredients:

- Cherry tomatoes
- Fresh mozzarella balls
- Fresh basil leaves
- Balsamic glaze (optional, for drizzling)
- Skewers

Instructions:

1. Thread a cherry tomato, a mozzarella ball, and a basil leaf onto each skewer.
2. Arrange skewers on a serving platter.
3. Optional: Drizzle with balsamic glaze before serving.

Nutrition Information:

- Calories: 60
- Protein: 4g
- Carbohydrates: 2g
- Fat: 4g
- Fiber: 1g
- Sugar: 1g
- Portion Size: 2 skewers

Spicy Roasted Cauliflower Bites

Ingredients:

- 1 head of cauliflower, cut into florets
- 2 tablespoons of olive oil
- 1 teaspoon of chili powder
- 1/2 teaspoon of garlic powder
- Salt and pepper to taste

Instructions:

1. Preheat oven to 425°F (220°C).
2. In a bowl, toss cauliflower florets with olive oil, chili powder, garlic powder, salt, and pepper.
3. Spread cauliflower in a single layer on a baking sheet.
4. Roast for 20-25 minutes until golden brown and crispy.
5. Serve hot.

Nutrition Information:

- Calories: 60
- Protein: 2g
- Carbohydrates: 5g
- Fat: 4g
- Fiber: 2g
- Sugar: 2g
- Portion Size: 1/2 cup of cauliflower bites

Avocado and Bean Dip

Ingredients:

- 1 ripe avocado
- 1 can of black beans, drained and rinsed
- 1 clove of garlic
- Juice of 1 lime
- Salt and pepper to taste

Instructions:

1. In a food processor, blend avocado, black beans, garlic, lime juice, salt, and pepper until smooth.
2. Serve with whole grain crackers or vegetable sticks.

Nutrition Information:

- Calories: 100
- Protein: 4g
- Carbohydrates: 10g
- Fat: 6g
- Fiber: 5g
- Sugar: 1g
- Portion Size: 1/4 cup of dip

Mini Quinoa Patties

Ingredients:

- 1 cup of cooked quinoa
- 1/4 cup of grated Parmesan cheese
- 1/4 cup of breadcrumbs
- 1 egg
- 2 tablespoons of chopped fresh herbs (such as parsley or cilantro)
- Salt and pepper to taste
- Olive oil for frying

Instructions:

1. In a bowl, mix cooked quinoa, Parmesan cheese, breadcrumbs, egg, chopped herbs, salt, and pepper.
2. Form mixture into small patties.
3. Heat olive oil in a skillet over medium heat.
4. Fry patties for 3-4 minutes on each side until golden brown.
5. Serve hot.

Nutrition Information:

- Calories: 80
- Protein: 4g
- Carbohydrates: 8g
- Fat: 4g

- Fiber: 1g

- Sugar: 0g

- Portion Size: 2 patties

Apple Slices with Almond Butter

Ingredients:

- 1 apple, sliced

- 2 tablespoons of almond butter

Instructions:

1. Spread almond butter on apple slices.

2. Serve as a tasty and nutritious snack.

Nutrition Information:

- Calories: 150

- Protein: 3g

- Carbohydrates: 15g

- Fat: 9g

- Fiber: 4g

- Sugar: 10g

- Portion Size: 1 medium apple with 2 tablespoons of almond butter

Zucchini Fritters

Ingredients:

- 2 medium zucchinis, grated
- 1/4 cup of grated Parmesan cheese
- 1/4 cup of breadcrumbs
- 1 egg
- 2 tablespoons of chopped fresh dill
- Salt and pepper to taste
- Olive oil for frying

Instructions:

1. Place grated zucchini in a clean kitchen towel and squeeze out excess moisture.
2. In a bowl, mix squeezed zucchini, Parmesan cheese, breadcrumbs, egg, chopped dill, salt, and pepper.
3. Form mixture into small patties.
4. Heat olive oil in a skillet over medium heat.
5. Fry fritters for 3-4 minutes on each side until golden brown.
6. Serve hot.

Nutrition Information:

- Calories: 90
- Protein: 4g
- Carbohydrates: 8g

- Fat: 5g

- Fiber: 2g

- Sugar: 3g

- Portion Size: 2 fritters

Chapter 6: Desserts

Indulging in desserts can be a delightful part of any meal, and with the right recipes, they can also be a nutritious addition to your diet. From rich chocolate treats to fruity delights, these desserts offer both flavor and health benefits. Each recipe is carefully crafted to provide a balance of nutrients while satisfying your sweet cravings.

Dark Chocolate Avocado Mousse

Ingredients:

- 2 ripe avocados
- 1/4 cup cocoa powder
- 1/4 cup maple syrup
- 1 teaspoon vanilla extract

Instructions:

1. Scoop the flesh of the avocados into a blender or food processor.
2. Add cocoa powder, maple syrup, and vanilla extract.
3. Blend until smooth and creamy.
4. Chill in the refrigerator for at least 30 minutes before serving.

Nutrition Information:

- Calories: 180
- Protein: 3g
- Carbohydrates: 15g
- Fat: 13g
- Fiber: 7g
- Sugar: 6g
- Portion Size: 1/2 cup

Baked Apples with Cinnamon

Ingredients:

- 4 apples, cored
- 2 tablespoons honey
- 1 teaspoon cinnamon

Instructions:

1. Preheat oven to 375°F (190°C).
2. Place cored apples in a baking dish.
3. Drizzle honey over the apples and sprinkle with cinnamon.
4. Bake for 25-30 minutes until apples are tender.
5. Serve warm.

Nutrition Information:

- Calories: 120
- Protein: 1g
- Carbohydrates: 32g
- Fat: 0g
- Fiber: 5g
- Sugar: 24g
- Portion Size: 1 apple

Chia Seed Pudding with Mango

Ingredients:

- 1/4 cup chia seeds
- 1 cup almond milk
- 1 tablespoon honey or maple syrup
- 1/2 teaspoon vanilla extract
- 1 ripe mango, diced

Instructions:

1. In a bowl, mix chia seeds, almond milk, honey or maple syrup, and vanilla extract.
2. Stir well and let it sit in the refrigerator for at least 2 hours or overnight.
3. Serve chilled, topped with diced mango.

Nutrition Information:

- Calories: 200
- Protein: 5g
- Carbohydrates: 25g
- Fat: 9g
- Fiber: 11g
- Sugar: 14g
- Portion Size: 1/2 cup

Berry and Greek Yogurt Parfait

Ingredients:

- 1 cup Greek yogurt
- 1/2 cup mixed berries (strawberries, blueberries, raspberries)
- 1/4 cup granola
- 1 tablespoon honey

Instructions:

1. In a glass or jar, layer Greek yogurt, mixed berries, and granola.
2. Drizzle with honey.
3. Repeat layers if desired.
4. Serve chilled.

Nutrition Information:

- Calories: 250
- Protein: 18g
- Carbohydrates: 35g
- Fat: 6g
- Fiber: 6g
- Sugar: 20g
- Portion Size: 1 cup

Almond Flour Brownies

Ingredients:

- 1 cup almond flour
- 1/2 cup cocoa powder
- 1/2 cup honey or maple syrup
- 1/4 cup coconut oil, melted
- 2 eggs
- 1 teaspoon vanilla extract
- 1/4 teaspoon baking soda
- Pinch of salt

Instructions:

1. Preheat oven to 350°F (175°C) and grease a baking dish.

2. In a bowl, mix almond flour, cocoa powder, honey or maple syrup, melted coconut oil, eggs, vanilla extract, baking soda, and salt until well combined.

3. Pour the batter into the prepared baking dish.

4. Bake for 20-25 minutes until the edges are set.

5. Allow to cool before slicing into squares.

Nutrition Information:

- Calories: 180

- Protein: 5g

- Carbohydrates: 15g

- Fat: 12g

- Fiber: 3g

- Sugar: 10g

- Portion Size: 1 brownie

Banana and Oat Cookies

Ingredients:

- 2 ripe bananas, mashed

- 1 1/2 cups rolled oats

- 1/4 cup almond butter

- 1/4 cup raisins or chocolate chips (optional)

- 1 teaspoon cinnamon

- Pinch of salt

Instructions:

1. Preheat oven to 350°F (175°C) and line a baking sheet with parchment paper.
2. In a bowl, mix mashed bananas, rolled oats, almond butter, raisins or chocolate chips (if using), cinnamon, and salt until well combined.
3. Drop spoonfuls of the dough onto the prepared baking sheet and flatten slightly with a fork.
4. Bake for 12-15 minutes until golden brown.
5. Allow to cool before serving.

Nutrition Information:

- Calories: 120
- Protein: 3g
- Carbohydrates: 20g
- Fat: 4g
- Fiber: 3g
- Sugar: 7g
- Portion Size: 2 cookies

Coconut Flour Chocolate Cake

Ingredients:

- 1/2 cup coconut flour
- 1/2 cup cocoa powder
- 1/2 cup honey or maple syrup
- 1/4 cup coconut oil, melted
- 6 eggs
- 1 teaspoon vanilla extract
- 1/2 teaspoon baking soda
- Pinch of salt

Instructions:

1. Preheat oven to 350°F (175°C) and grease a cake pan.
2. In a bowl, mix coconut flour, cocoa powder, honey or maple syrup, melted coconut oil, eggs, vanilla extract, baking soda, and salt until smooth.
3. Pour the batter into the prepared cake pan.
4. Bake for 25-30 minutes until a toothpick inserted into the center comes out clean.
5. Allow to cool before slicing and serving.

Nutrition Information:

- Calories: 180
- Protein: 6g

- Carbohydrates: 20g
- Fat: 10g
- Fiber: 5g
- Sugar: 12g
- Portion Size: 1 slice

Mixed Berry Crumble

Ingredients:

- 2 cups mixed berries (strawberries, blueberries, raspberries)
- 1/2 cup almond flour
- 1/4 cup oats
- 1/4 cup honey or maple syrup
- 2 tablespoons coconut oil, melted
- 1 teaspoon cinnamon
- Pinch of salt

Instructions:

1. Preheat oven to 350°F (175°C) and grease a baking dish.
2. In a bowl, mix mixed berries with 2 tablespoons of honey or maple syrup. Spread the berries evenly in the prepared baking dish.

3. In another bowl, combine almond flour, oats, remaining honey or maple syrup, melted coconut oil, cinnamon, and salt until crumbly.

4. Sprinkle the crumble mixture over the berries.

5. Bake for 25-30 minutes until the topping is golden brown and the berries are bubbling.

6. Allow to cool slightly before serving.

Nutrition Information:

- Calories: 220
- Protein: 4g
- Carbohydrates: 30g
- Fat: 10g
- Fiber: 6g
- Sugar: 18g
- Portion Size: 1/2 cup

Frozen Yogurt Bark with Berries

Ingredients:

- 2 cups Greek yogurt
- 1/4 cup honey or maple syrup
- 1 teaspoon vanilla extract
- 1 cup mixed berries (strawberries, blueberries, raspberries)

Instructions:

1. In a bowl, mix Greek yogurt, honey or maple syrup, and vanilla extract until smooth.
2. Line a baking sheet with parchment paper.
3. Spread the yogurt mixture evenly onto the parchment paper.
4. Sprinkle mixed berries over the yogurt.
5. Place the baking sheet in the freezer for at least 2 hours until firm.
6. Once frozen, break the yogurt bark into pieces.
7. Serve immediately as a refreshing treat.

Nutrition Information:

- Calories: 120
- Protein: 8g
- Carbohydrates: 20g
- Fat: 2g
- Fiber: 2g
- Sugar: 15g
- Portion Size: 1/2 cup

Apple Cinnamon Muffins

Ingredients:

- 2 cups almond flour

- 1 teaspoon baking powder

- 1/2 teaspoon baking soda

- 1/4 teaspoon salt

- 1 tablespoon cinnamon

- 2 eggs

- 1/4 cup honey or maple syrup

- 1/4 cup coconut oil, melted

- 1 cup grated apple (about 2 apples)

- 1/4 cup chopped walnuts (optional)

Instructions:

1. Preheat oven to 350°F (175°C) and line a muffin tin with liners.

2. In a large bowl, whisk together almond flour, baking powder, baking soda, salt, and cinnamon.

3. In another bowl, whisk together eggs, honey or maple syrup, and melted coconut oil.

4. Add the wet ingredients to the dry ingredients and mix until just combined.

5. Fold in grated apple and chopped walnuts (if using).

6. Divide the batter evenly among the muffin cups.

7. Bake for 20-25 minutes until a toothpick inserted into the center comes out clean.

8. Allow to cool before serving.

Nutrition Information:

- Calories: 180
- Protein: 5g
- Carbohydrates: 15g
- Fat: 12g
- Fiber: 3g
- Sugar: 8g
- Portion Size: 1 muffin

Carrot Cake Energy Balls

Ingredients:

- 1 cup rolled oats
- 1/2 cup shredded carrots
- 1/4 cup almond butter
- 1/4 cup honey or maple syrup
- 1/4 cup chopped walnuts
- 1 teaspoon cinnamon
- 1/2 teaspoon vanilla extract
- Pinch of salt

Instructions:

1. In a food processor, pulse rolled oats until they form a coarse flour-like consistency.

2. Add shredded carrots, almond butter, honey or maple syrup, chopped walnuts, cinnamon, vanilla extract, and salt.

3. Pulse until well combined and the mixture starts to stick together.

4. Roll the mixture into small balls using your hands.

5. Place the energy balls on a baking sheet lined with parchment paper.

6. Chill in the refrigerator for at least 30 minutes before serving.

Nutrition Information:

- Calories: 120
- Protein: 3g
- Carbohydrates: 15g
- Fat: 6g
- Fiber: 2g
- Sugar: 8g
- Portion Size: 1 energy ball

Peach Sorbet

Ingredients:

- 2 cups frozen peaches
- 1/4 cup coconut water or almond milk

- 1 tablespoon honey or maple syrup (optional)
- Juice of 1/2 lemon (optional)

Instructions:

1. In a blender or food processor, combine frozen peaches, coconut water or almond milk, honey or maple syrup (if using), and lemon juice (if using).
2. Blend until smooth and creamy, scraping down the sides as needed.
3. Serve immediately as soft-serve sorbet or transfer to a container and freeze for a firmer texture.
4. Allow to soften slightly before scooping and serving.

Nutrition Information:

- Calories: 80
- Protein: 1g
- Carbohydrates: 20g
- Fat: 0g
- Fiber: 2g
- Sugar: 16g
- Portion Size: 1/2 cup

Sugar-Free Lemon Bars

Ingredients:

- 1 cup almond flour
- 1/4 cup coconut flour
- 1/4 cup coconut oil, melted
- 3 tablespoons lemon juice
- Zest of 1 lemon
- 2 tablespoons honey or maple syrup (optional)
- 4 eggs
- 1/2 teaspoon baking powder
- Pinch of salt

Instructions:

1. Preheat oven to 350°F (175°C) and line a baking dish with parchment paper.
2. In a bowl, mix almond flour, coconut flour, melted coconut oil, lemon juice, lemon zest, and honey or maple syrup (if using) until a dough forms.
3. Press the dough evenly into the bottom of the prepared baking dish.
4. Bake for 12-15 minutes until lightly golden.
5. Meanwhile, in another bowl, whisk together eggs, baking powder, and salt until well combined.
6. Pour the egg mixture over the baked crust.

7. Return to the oven and bake for an additional 15-20 minutes until the filling is set.

8. Allow to cool before slicing into bars.

Nutrition Information:

- Calories: 120
- Protein: 5g
- Carbohydrates: 10g
- Fat: 8g
- Fiber: 2g
- Sugar: 2g
- Portion Size: 1 bar

Pumpkin Spice Bites

Ingredients:

- 1 cup rolled oats
- 1/2 cup pumpkin puree
- 1/4 cup almond butter
- 2 tablespoons honey or maple syrup
- 1 teaspoon pumpkin pie spice
- 1/2 teaspoon vanilla extract
- Pinch of salt

Instructions:

1. In a food processor, pulse rolled oats until they form a coarse flour-like consistency.
2. Add pumpkin puree, almond butter, honey or maple syrup, pumpkin pie spice, vanilla extract, and salt.
3. Pulse until well combined and the mixture starts to stick together.
4. Roll the mixture into small bites using your hands.
5. Optional: Roll the bites in shredded coconut or chopped nuts for extra flavor.
6. Place the bites on a baking sheet lined with parchment paper.
7. Chill in the refrigerator for at least 30 minutes before serving.

Nutrition Information:

- Calories: 100
- Protein: 3g
- Carbohydrates: 15g
- Fat: 4g
- Fiber: 2g
- Sugar: 5g
- Portion Size: 2 bites

Dark Chocolate Dipped Strawberries

Ingredients:

- 1 pint fresh strawberries, washed and dried
- 4 ounces dark chocolate, chopped
- 1 teaspoon coconut oil

Instructions:

1. Line a baking sheet with parchment paper.
2. In a microwave-safe bowl, combine chopped dark chocolate and coconut oil.
3. Microwave in 30-second intervals, stirring in between, until the chocolate is melted and smooth.
4. Holding each strawberry by the stem, dip it into the melted chocolate, coating about two-thirds of the berry.
5. Place the dipped strawberries onto the prepared baking sheet.
6. Optional: Sprinkle with chopped nuts or shredded coconut before the chocolate sets.
7. Place the baking sheet in the refrigerator for 15-20 minutes until the chocolate is set.
8. Serve chilled as a decadent dessert or snack.

Nutrition Information:

- Calories: 50

- Protein: 1g
- Carbohydrates: 7g
- Fat: 3g
- Fiber: 2g
- Sugar: 4g
- Portion Size: 2 strawberries

Chapter 7: Smoothies

Smoothies are a fantastic way to pack a variety of nutrients into a single, delicious drink. For individuals managing type 2 diabetes, smoothies can offer a convenient way to incorporate fruits, vegetables, and other healthful ingredients into their diets.

Green Detox Smoothie

Ingredients:

- 1 cup spinach
- 1/2 cup cucumber, chopped
- 1 green apple, chopped
- 1/2 lemon, juiced
- 1 cup water
- 1 tsp grated ginger

Instructions:

1. Add all ingredients to a blender.
2. Blend until smooth.
3. Serve immediately.

Nutrition Information (per serving):

- Calories: 80

- Protein: 1g

- Carbohydrates: 20g

- Fat: 0g

- Fiber: 4g

- Sugar: 10g

- Portion size: 1 glass

Berry Banana Smoothie

Ingredients:

- 1/2 banana

- 1/2 cup strawberries

- 1/2 cup blueberries

- 1 cup almond milk

- 1 tbsp chia seeds

Instructions:

1. Combine all ingredients in a blender.

2. Blend until creamy.

3. Pour into a glass and enjoy.

Nutrition Information (per serving):

- Calories: 150

- Protein: 3g

- Carbohydrates: 30g

- Fat: 4g

- Fiber: 7g

- Sugar: 15g

- Portion size: 1 glass

Tropical Mango Smoothie

Ingredients:

- 1 cup mango chunks

- 1/2 banana

- 1/2 cup pineapple chunks

- 1 cup coconut water

Instructions:

1. Place all ingredients in a blender.
2. Blend until smooth and creamy.
3. Serve chilled.

Nutrition Information (per serving):

- Calories: 140

- Protein: 2g

- Carbohydrates: 35g

- Fat: 0g

- Fiber: 3g

- Sugar: 30g

- Portion size: 1 glass

Spinach and Kale Smoothie

Ingredients:

- 1 cup spinach

- 1/2 cup kale

- 1/2 banana

- 1/2 cup apple juice

- 1/2 cup water

Instructions:

1. Combine all ingredients in a blender.

2. Blend until smooth.

3. Serve immediately.

Nutrition Information (per serving):

- Calories: 90

- Protein: 2g

- Carbohydrates: 22g

- Fat: 0g

- Fiber: 4g

- Sugar: 14g
- Portion size: 1 glass

Peanut Butter and Banana Smoothie

Ingredients:

- 1 banana
- 1 tbsp peanut butter
- 1 cup almond milk
- 1 tsp honey (optional)

Instructions:

1. Add all ingredients to a blender.
2. Blend until creamy.
3. Serve immediately.

Nutrition Information (per serving):

- Calories: 220
- Protein: 5g
- Carbohydrates: 30g
- Fat: 9g
- Fiber: 4g
- Sugar: 15g
- Portion size: 1 glass

Avocado and Berry Smoothie

Ingredients:

- 1/2 avocado
- 1/2 cup mixed berries
- 1/2 banana
- 1 cup almond milk

Instructions:

1. Place all ingredients in a blender.
2. Blend until smooth.
3. Serve chilled.

Nutrition Information (per serving):

- Calories: 200
- Protein: 3g
- Carbohydrates: 26g
- Fat: 10g
- Fiber: 8g
- Sugar: 10g
- Portion size: 1 glass

Carrot Ginger Smoothie

Ingredients:

- 1 cup carrot juice
- 1/2 cup orange juice
- 1/2 banana
- 1 tsp grated ginger

Instructions:

1. Add all ingredients to a blender.
2. Blend until smooth.
3. Serve immediately.

Nutrition Information (per serving):

- Calories: 110
- Protein: 1g
- Carbohydrates: 25g
- Fat: 0g
- Fiber: 3g
- Sugar: 16g
- Portion size: 1 glass

Pineapple and Spinach Smoothie

Ingredients:

- 1 cup spinach
- 1/2 cup pineapple chunks
- 1/2 banana
- 1 cup coconut water

Instructions:

1. Combine all ingredients in a blender.
2. Blend until smooth.
3. Serve immediately.

Nutrition Information (per serving):

- Calories: 100
- Protein: 1g
- Carbohydrates: 25g
- Fat: 0g
- Fiber: 2g
- Sugar: 20g
- Portion size: 1 glass

Almond Butter and Berry Smoothie

Ingredients:

- 1/2 cup mixed berries
- 1 tbsp almond butter
- 1/2 banana
- 1 cup almond milk

Instructions:

1. Add all ingredients to a blender.
2. Blend until creamy.
3. Serve immediately.

Nutrition Information (per serving):

- Calories: 180
- Protein: 4g
- Carbohydrates: 25g
- Fat: 8g
- Fiber: 5g
- Sugar: 14g
- Portion size: 1 glass

Beetroot and Berry Smoothie

Ingredients:

- 1/2 cup beetroot, cooked and chopped
- 1/2 cup mixed berries
- 1/2 banana
- 1 cup water

Instructions:

1. Place all ingredients in a blender.
2. Blend until smooth.
3. Serve chilled.

Nutrition Information (per serving):

- Calories: 110
- Protein: 2g
- Carbohydrates: 26g
- Fat: 0g
- Fiber: 5g
- Sugar: 18g
- Portion size: 1 glass

Coconut and Pineapple Smoothie

Ingredients:

- 1/2 cup pineapple chunks
- 1/2 cup coconut milk
- 1/2 banana
- 1 cup water

Instructions:

1. Add all ingredients to a blender.
2. Blend until smooth.
3. Serve immediately.

Nutrition Information (per serving):

- Calories: 130
- Protein: 1g
- Carbohydrates: 25g
- Fat: 4g
- Fiber: 3g
- Sugar: 18g
- Portion size: 1 glass

Cucumber and Mint Smoothie

Ingredients:

- 1 cup cucumber, chopped
- 1/2 cup mint leaves
- 1/2 banana
- 1 cup water
- 1 tsp lemon juice

Instructions:

1. Combine all ingredients in a blender.
2. Blend until smooth.
3. Serve chilled.

Nutrition Information (per serving):

- Calories: 70
- Protein: 1g
- Carbohydrates: 18g
- Fat: 0g
- Fiber: 3g
- Sugar: 10g
- Portion size: 1 glass

Apple Pie Smoothie

Ingredients:

- 1 apple, chopped
- 1/2 banana
- 1/2 cup oats
- 1/2 tsp cinnamon
- 1 cup almond milk

Instructions:

1. Add all ingredients to a blender.
2. Blend until smooth.
3. Serve immediately.

Nutrition Information (per serving):

- Calories: 180
- Protein: 3g
- Carbohydrates: 35g
- Fat: 3g
- Fiber: 6g
- Sugar: 16g
- Portion size: 1 glass

Pumpkin Spice Smoothie

Ingredients:

- 1/2 cup pumpkin puree
- 1/2 banana
- 1/2 tsp pumpkin spice
- 1 cup almond milk
- 1 tsp honey (optional)

Instructions:

1. Combine all ingredients in a blender.
2. Blend until smooth.
3. Serve chilled.

Nutrition Information (per serving):

- Calories: 130
- Protein: 2g
- Carbohydrates: 30g
- Fat: 2g
- Fiber: 5g
- Sugar: 14g
- Portion size: 1 glass

Kiwi and Kale Smoothie

Ingredients:

- 1 kiwi, peeled and chopped
- 1 cup kale
- 1/2 banana
- 1 cup water
- 1 tsp honey (optional)

Instructions:

1. Place all ingredients in a blender.
2. Blend until smooth.
3. Serve immediately.

Nutrition Information (per serving):

- Calories: 80
- Protein: 2g
- Carbohydrates: 20g
- Fat: 0g
- Fiber: 4g
- Sugar: 10g
- Portion size: 1 glass

CONCLUSION

As we conclude "Quick and Healthy Vegetarian Meals for Type 2 Diabetes," it's essential to reflect on the journey we've undertaken through this book. The primary aim was to equip you with the knowledge, tools, and inspiration to manage your diabetes effectively while enjoying a delicious, nutritious, and varied vegetarian diet.

Throughout this book, we've explored the critical role that diet plays in managing type 2 diabetes. By focusing on plant-based meals, we've highlighted how a vegetarian diet can provide ample nutrients, help maintain stable blood sugar levels, and support overall health. The recipes and meal plans provided are not just designed to be diabetes-friendly but also to be quick, convenient, and flavorful, ensuring that you can easily integrate them into your daily routine.

Final Thoughts:
Adopting a vegetarian diet to manage type 2 diabetes is not just a temporary dietary change but a lifestyle choice that can lead to long-term health benefits. The variety of recipes and meal plans in this book are designed to be sustainable and enjoyable, making it easier to adhere to a healthy eating plan.

Remember, the journey to managing diabetes effectively is a continuous process that involves regular monitoring, consultation with healthcare professionals, and making informed food choices. By incorporating the recipes and tips provided in this book into your daily life, you are taking a significant step towards better health and well-being.

We hope this book serves as a valuable resource and inspiration for you to embrace a healthier, vegetarian lifestyle that supports your diabetes management. Here's to delicious meals, better health, and a fulfilling life.